ADRENAL FATIGUE

Fighting the Root of Systemic Stupor, Tension, and Misery

Second Edition

Leah Olsen

© 2016

Adrenal Fatigue – Second Edition

©Copyright 2016

Disclaimer

The information provided in this book is designed to provide helpful information on the subjects discussed. The author's books are only meant to provide the reader with the basics knowledge of the topic in question, without any warranties regarding whether the reader will, or will not, be able to incorporate and apply all the information provided. Although the writer will make his best effort share her insights, the topic in question is a complex one, and each person needs a different timeframe to fully incorporate new information. Neither this book, nor any of the author's books constitute a promise that the reader will learn anything within a certain timeframe.

Table of Contents

Introduction:

The stillness of the room was broken by the high pitched sound of the wake up timer signifying another day has arrived. It was sufficiently noisy to horrendously wake you up from your sweet and unquenchable sleep. The jolting cry of the signal has spoiled your first cognizant seconds. However the prior night you hit the sack, you expected to set the volume at full force. You have to wake up or you'll be late for work.

The wake up timer continued crying in your ears, making each snapshot of your vain endeavors for expanded rest painfully discomforting. When you succeeded pulling the gigantic weight of your body off from the comfortable bed, you were all the while yawning for the fourth time. Going after the end table appeared a genuine annoyance. You have irately put the wake up timer out of its hopelessness with a pummel of your palm against the catch.

You are currently towing your feet in each of the seven stages to the apparently interminable separation towards the lavatory. The weight of two planets was on your shoulders until icy water from the shower jarred you wide conscious, just to acknowledge despite everything you're wearing your dozing outfit. At that point you wiped yourself dry, spruced up, and quickly left the house. You begin your 8:00 AM shift at 9:00 AM.

The pressure faded away, alongside your diminishing vitality, almost an hour subsequent to getting a tirade of censures from your predominant. Crossed by the before encounter, you are in no inclination for amenities or casual banter from your colleagues. Once home, you thought your day would never deteriorate. Nothing in the TV appeared to be intriguing. Perusing the pages of your most loved book couldn't start a shred of excitement that will help you overlook how awful your day went. Overwhelming trance, negative pressure, and the enduring dejection were the glaring highlighted subtle elements of your day.

Upon reading the introduction, let me ask you something. Do you see yourself in that battle? Have you encountered this yourself? Did the same account look somewhat like your regular reality? Do you happen to know other individuals who, possibly, may have been encountering this sort of battle firsthand? At first look, the chain of occasions outlined in the past sections appeared like a kind "awful day" – nothing that a container of lager and giggling couldn't without much of a stretch cure.

Tragically, if the same hopeless cycle has repeated for a month or more, there's a tremendous shot that a man is experiencing a much genuine issue. It might be helpful for standard individuals to charge this to straightforward lethargy. An all the more perceiving yet detached individual would presume that the tenacious "nonappearance of life" is a fundamental emotional instability, exacerbated because of an uncertain traumatic affair. Be that as it may, a great many people would not have effectively thought about how possible it is of a man's entire general wretchedness being created by a disappointment in the inward organs.

It's hard to believe, but it's true. This organic issue that leaves a man physically, mentally and sincerely down while showing up totally unscathed is scandalously called "adrenal fatigue". In this book, you will take in all the appropriate bits of data expected to manage this sort of shrewd ailment. Thinking about adrenal fatigue is the initial phase in fighting it.

Chapter 1:
Basic Bio 101

Keeping in mind the end goal to pick up a full comprehension of adrenal fatigue, it is critical to make sense of what capacities the adrenaline plays in the human body. Before the cutting edge times, there has been little appreciation in regards to the exceptional way of adrenals. The advancements in the field of human science have taken incredible walks over a couple of eras, permitting medicinal science to step by step disentangle the secrets of the adrenals. Henceforth, whatever will be talked about in this part depends on a rearranged review of the uncommon field of endocrinology.

Adrenal Glands

All animals in the set of all animals have adrenal glands, notwithstanding including strong single-cell life forms. It makes sense that individuals likewise have these vital organs. The adrenal glands are a couple of triangular-shaped organs that create key hormones that permitted every inward organ to work effectively.

It is imperative to observe that until the revelation of the 15th Century Italian scholar named Bartolomeo Esutachi, mankind has no earlier learning of adrenaline glands. He was one of only a handful couple of researchers credited for the foundation of human life structures as an imperative branch of organic review. Beside the kidneys, Bartolomeo Eustachi was additionally credited for the detailed analysis of the structure of vital organs like the ear, the heart, the brain, and the spinal cord.

Inquisitively, the word adrenaline is gotten from a blend of two Latin terminologies. The word *ad* signifies "close" and the word *renes* interprets as "kidneys". This essentially clarifies their correct area in the human body, sitting on top of the two organs in charge for filtering residue wastes from the circulatory framework.

Each of the adrenaline glands has a standard estimation of 3 inches long and 1.5 inches tall. In the event that one needs to make a relative layman examination, the adrenaline glands take after an oak seed or walnut as far as its normal size. A solitary adrenaline glands measures a normal of 4 grams. To the extent their appearance is concerned, both of these glands are moderately one of a kind from each other. The left adrenaline gland resembles a bended mass, taking after either a wide club or a sporadic sickle. The right adrenaline gland bears a nearby closeness with a hill. Every match of glands is included two different parts.

The adrenal cortex is the external part of the organ that produces hormones that assume an essential part in the inward framework. This external part of the adrenaline glands makes *cortisol*, a protein that directs digestion system. Another key biochemical part delivered by the adrenal cortex is the *aldosterone*, which is principally in charge of controlling the body's circulatory strain.

The adrenal medulla is the internal part of the gland that is in charge of delivering hormones that are categorized as unnecessary. Strangely, still, the key hormones released by the inside adrenaline gland contained the namesake *adrenaline*. In a straightforward definition, the adrenaline empowers the body to adapt up to stressors. Strangely, the adrenal medulla just contains 10 percent of the aggregate scope for each of the adrenaline gland's structure.

Anatomical Physiology

As said before, the fundamental reasons for the adrenaline glands are to manage the body and empower it to adapt with anxiety. It is vital to consider the way that both capacities are reliant with each other. At the end of the day, the body can't balance out its general operations in the event that it can't oversee nervousness. Moreover, the body can't conquer injury if its tissues and organs are weak.

With that reality basically settled, the time has come to investigate another critical question concerning the adrenaline glands - How precisely does the adrenaline glands function?

Mostly, the adrenaline glands decide the body's "battle or flight reaction". It is critical to perceive the all-inclusive actuality that the human body is continually barraged with weight from a wide assortment of sources. Stressors may incorporate wounds, contaminations, and even negative passionate responses like tension, temper, and trouble. Despite how one would intentionally respond when he or she experiences an upsetting knowledge, the fundamental motivation behind the adrenaline organs is to keep the body from totally coming up short.

As specified earlier, hormones like the cortisol are in charge of directing the body's digestion system. Referred to all the more regularly as a "stress hormones", the cortisol and aldosterone direct digestion system and control circulatory strain by playing out the accompanying particular physiological responses:

They quicken the body's utilization of carbohydrates and fats.

They viably change over fats and proteins into energy.

They upgrade the best possible dissemination of stored fats.

They adjust the glucose levels.

They increment the execution of the central nervous system.

They enhance the body's immune reactions.

They enhance the body's anti-inflammatory activities.

They upgrade the body's general cardiovascular execution.

They alter the general gastrointestinal progression.

These particular physiological alterations empower the human body to react all the more fittingly at whatever point it is faced with stressors. There is an extensive variety of improved accomplishments at whatever point the adrenaline organs enact its flight or battle guard instrument.

A standout amongst the most emphatically got illustrations is best shown in unpleasant angry situations. Picture a slight asthmatic young kid getting away or guarding oneself from a little gathering of school spooks. A very working pair of adrenaline glands will enact its assortment of physiological responses so as to incline one's body as per the particular requests important to play out a particular arrangement of activities. In the event that the casualty chooses to escape, he will run quicker and encounter a transient increment of stamina due to an abruptly improved cardiovascular execution. In the event that the casualty chooses to battle back, the successful utilization of vitality and dispersion of supplements in the framework will permit him to toss all the more capable and exact strikes and in addition adequately square or dodge an adversary's hit due to increased reflexes. In any case, the apparently innocuous individual changes into a very working hostile because of a brilliant match of adrenaline organs.

In the particular situation portrayed above, passionate uneasiness and pressure kick off the adrenaline glands. This trigger empowers the adrenaline glands to give a support in one's physical execution. In any case, it is imperative to observe that the recurrence of good adrenal reaction is less predictable than one may anticipate. There are times when stress overpowers the characteristic battle or flight reaction. At the point when this happens, the poor asthmatic young kid unfortunately gets another disagreeable round of physical or mental manhandle from his tormentors.

Adrenal Checks and Balance

The past subchapter presumed that the adrenaline framework may now and then experience a breakdown. At the point when thinking about the prior situation, one can without much of a stretch charge the inability to adapt up to worry as "one stroke of misfortune". In any case, there is a clearer comprehension of why the nature of the body's general execution is lessened. The motivation behind why the adrenaline glands some of the time don't work well as far as adapting up to stress is that there is close to nothing or a lot of the "stress hormones" discharged by the organs. It makes sense that the arrival of cortisol must follow the adequate volume and term.

These are the accompanying impacts of having an abundance of cortisol as far as both length and general amount:

The body will have expanded stomach fat. It makes sense that the amplification of the waistline is frequently connected with genuine medical issues

13

coming about because of large amounts of bad cholesterol.

The body will encounter hyperglycemia, or all the more regularly known as "sugar rush". Therefore, an individual may encounter restlessness and impeded (sporadic) thought-handling. Eventually, this will wind up in a "sugar crash" and the individual will feel extraordinary fatigue.

The body will have an expanded circulatory strain, for which an individual may encounter unsteadiness, best case scenario, and additionally vertigo and headache even from a pessimistic standpoint.

The body will have a diminished muscle mass (muscle atrophy). Thus, the individual is more probable at danger of having cardiovascular sicknesses because of an overabundance of fats. All things considered, muscle piece practically decides a tremendous part of a human body's general wellness. Low muscle mass additionally results to the slower recuperating procedure of an open injury.

The body will have a diminished bone thickness. Aside from the undeniable laziness coming about because of this illness, an individual has a higher danger of bone breaks because of a generally minor limit injury.

Besides, the impacts of having a low cortisol incorporate the accompanying:

The body will encounter fatigue, especially amid hours of the day when vitality levels are at its peak (e.g. morning and late morning).

The body will encounter hypoglycemia. This glucose imbalance causes the person to wind up distinctly cranky, lazy and discouraged. The indications very take after a wide scope of gentle starvation.

The body will have a diminished circulatory strain. Much the same as hypertension, low circulatory strain causes tipsiness, queasiness and fall from serious depletion best case scenario.

The body will endure irritations. Subsequently, an individual will probably have swelling and skin injuries because of gentle hypersensitivities and other resistant triggers.

At last, both end of the range bargains the accompanying parts of life:

Nature of rest

Level of cognizance

Level of insusceptibility from diseases

Chapter 2:
Patient History

The past part talked about various key focuses to consider regarding understanding the nature and qualities of the adrenaline glands. Beside its disclosure in the 15th Century, next to no is ever comprehended about them until the 21st Century. Through cutting edge pharmaceutical, the adrenaline glands are thought to be the wellspring of a biochemical way of dealing with stress against stress. What's more, much the same as other vital organs in the body, the adrenaline glands are likewise, best case scenario, inclined to breakdown and, at the very least, add up to disappointment.

This part of the book is committed to comprehension the key focuses that clarify how adrenaline glands fall flat. In this part, you won't just find the historical backdrop of adrenal fatigue as an analysis in present day pharmaceutical. You will even figure out how to speculate whether or not "your" adrenaline glands are in a terrible shape. Take note: the data you may gather viewing manifestations just serve as a general reference. As usual, it is exceptionally fitting to look for legitimate therapeutic examination for the total assurance of one's general physical state.

Chronology

Addison's Disease

The main solid review concerning the disappointment of adrenaline organs can be followed back in the 1800's. The 19th Century English doctor named Dr. Thomas Addison exhibited his historic medicinal research in the South London Medical Society in 1849. As indicated by his proposition, the "general condition of anemia episode to grown-up guys" indicated the debilitated adrenaline glands as the wellspring of comparative manifestations predominant in the assortment of corresponded case reports (e.g. low vitality, feeble invulnerable framework, and so on.). From that point on, this handicap was known as the Addison's Disease, courtesy of its pioneer.

Swine Serum

Taking after Dr. Addison's revelation of the previously mentioned endocrinal sickness, doctors have practically committed a generous exertion in comprehension and curing this disease. Be that as it may, the main most noteworthy type of treatment did not surface until 1898. The Canadian doctor (and one of the two soonest pioneers of cutting edge drug's "residency program) named Sir William Osler made a treatment for the Addison's Disease utilizing the adrenal cells from a pig. It is imperative to observe that, regardless of the numerous triumphs in Dr. Osler's endeavors in pushing present day restorative practice to awesome statures, his porcine treatment practically hit a deadlock. Luckily, future eras of doctors would enhance the adrenal concentrate plot for drug.

The Schism

Assist advancements as far as understanding this field of endocrinology have brought about a partition among therapeutic defenders in the 20th Century. As time goes by over the span of the new rush of medicinal examinations, the polarization of the widespread agreement gets clearer. Some therapeutic defenders have added to the emergence of the conclusion called hypoadrenia - a more old term for adrenal fatigue.

In 1919, an Italian medical educator named Nicola Pende has cleared up what hypoadrenia is. As per him, this sickness is portrayed by a lopsidedness of hormones frequently ascribed to mellow or dormant states of the endocrine glands. This, among numerous different supports, were dismisses by spoilers who are persuaded that lone a detectable (physical) deformity in the general endocrine glands.

Accreditation Failure

Since the mid 1900's, diagnosing hypoadrenia has turned out to be hazardous. Since there is no test that can precisely analyze apparently generous or idle adrenal imperfection, any investigation will be viewed as arguable. On the off chance that there is one thing that demonstrates confounded in the field of drug, it is the component of vulnerability. From 1920's to 1940's, the uncertified therapeutic suppositions relating to adrenal fatigue have not infiltrated canon medical practice. Similarly, any types of treatment were respected with an equivalent level of suspicion (if not by and large objection). It would require a more drawn out investment before a lot of consideration is stood to this specific subject.

Renegade Doctors

Medical supporters of hypoadrenia or adrenal fatigue did not encounter a leap forward until the 1990's. Amid this time, an American doctor named Dr. James Wilson has figured out how to break down adrenal fatigue with a generous level of precision. A standout amongst the most powerful strategies that add to Dr. Wilson's work is the spit cortisol testing. Different doctors that encouraged the consciousness of adrenal fatigue in contemporary prescription incorporate specifically Dr. Richard Shames, Dr. Christiane Northrup and Dr. Michael Lam.

Unluckily, even with the battle of respectable doctors like Dr. Wilson, there still remains a solid restriction to adrenal fatigue as a positive therapeutic determination. It is one of the numerous particular situations where the standard medicinal group all in all remaining parts undecided, in spite of the developing prominence and acknowledgment in the lay society.

Survey Quiz

Instituting the expression "adrenal fatigue", Dr. James Wilson has additionally made it feasible for non-doctors to get a generally decent supposition of one's therapeutic condition. The Burnout Questionnaire is gone for giving a normal evaluation that decides "regardless of whether you are experiencing adrenal fatigue". Note: in spite of the conclusion derived by the consequence of the survey, it is still profoundly prudent to look for appropriate restorative counsel to decide the correct ailment, degree of the protest and the best possible game-plan to address the ailment.

Here is the rundown of inquiries, each to be appraised 0 to 5 (with 5 being the best esteem) regarding power:

- Do you tire more easily?
- Do you feel exhausted more than lively?
- Do you get aggravated when individuals let you know, "you don't look so great of late"?
- Are you working harder however finishing less?
- Are you progressively critical and upset?
- Do you regularly encounter mental suffering?
- Do you much of the time overlook due dates, arrangements, and individual things?
- Have you get to be distinctly touchier?
- Are you all the more crotchety?
- Are you baffled by individuals around you?
- Are you seeing your family members and close friends less often?
- Does doing a little routine undertaking (e.g. perusing reports, sending short cards to companions and making imperative calls) excessively boisterous in your timetable?
- Do you experience an increase in a number of physical complaints (e.g. muscle or joint aches, headaches, lingering colds and/or flu, etc.)?

o   Do you encounter an expansion in various physical grumblings (e.g. muscle or joint hurts, cerebral pains, waiting colds as well as influenza, and so on.)?
o   Is happiness an elusive idea and/or experience?
o   Are you not able to snicker or jab fun at yourself?
o   Does sex appear like a more troublesome act than pleasurable?
o   Do you have next to no to state to other individuals?

In the wake of demonstrating the numbers in every question, you need to figure the normal score ("total sum" divided by "the total number of questions"). The outcome will translate your rough diagnosis. The elucidation of the outcomes is as per the following:

0 to 25:   The individual doing fine.

26 to 35: The individual's anxiety is beginning to show.

36 to 50: The individual is a possibility for burnout

51 to 65: The individual is extremely wore out

Over 65: The individual is hazardously depleted

With the ailment being called adrenal fatigue, there is a justifiable reason motivation behind why Dr. Wilson utilized depletion as a dependable connection. Besides the conspicuous feeling of the compound thing "adrenal fatigue", debility (e.g. physical, enthusiastic and mental) for all intents and purposes incorporates each possible therapeutic conclusion concerning the human

21

condition. Nonetheless, the Burnout Questionnaire just gives a preparatory level of investigation.

Symptoms

There's something else entirely with adrenal fatigue than what was exhibited in the two past parts of the section. To the extent the depreciators are concerned, adrenal fatigue is basically a false ailment. Many have indicated its wide (and conceivably uncertain) side effects as the wellspring of adrenal fatigue's faulty determination. Be that as it may, what are the genuine manifestations connected with this dubious sickness?

Before getting further into that, it is vital to consider the way that adrenal fatigue as a sickness depends on a specific primary concern logical hypothesis. As indicated by Dr. Wilson; physical, mental and passionate fatigue can be conceivably created by the failure of the adrenaline glands to deliver the appropriate measure of cortisol. Given that start, adrenal fatigue is some way or another supported by these taking after physical pointers:

Symptom #1.
Inconvenience getting up.

Symptom #2.
Unending tiredness even in the wake of getting up in the morning.

Symptom #3.

Inconvenience thinking straight or finishing an errand.

These are only the most punctual signs that may advance into something genuine. Much the same as other degenerative diseases like cancer and Alzheimer's Disease, adrenal fatigue can form into a more genuine adaptation of its underlying finding. Note: additional data about Stages of Adrenal Fatigue will be talked about in Chapter 3 of the volume.

Chapter 3:
Second Opinion

The past parts of the book for the most part talked about the general way of adrenaline glands and its anxiety hormones, and a preparatory foundation on adrenal fatigue as an ailment. As specified in the past section, adrenal fatigue is a troublesome disease to close. There is something else entirely to the resolved suspicion of depreciators with regards to the issue with diagnosing hypoadrenia. In this current volume's section, you will have the capacity to take a stand and shape your own particular decision with respect to the dubious faction between two medical schools of thought concerning the fatigue contention.

Faux Diagnosis

The most predominant test of distinguishing adrenal fatigue is that this sort of disease takes after a wide assortment of clutters as far as the manifestations alone. As said in the past section, an underlying examination is constrained to the three wide signs. Ceaseless tiredness, absence of fixation and the failure to get up from bed are essentially a futile arrangement of criteria that, alone, couldn't give an indisputable examination without higher succeeding levels of physical review (e.g. audit of patient history, cortisol lab test, and broad perception).

Ruling Out: Level One

The three previously mentioned particular exhaustion manifestations can show in other basic however inconsequential illnesses. These scatters incorporate paleness, joint inflammation, diabetes, thyroid issues and heart disappointment. In any case, finishing up these different ailments can even be excessively hurried. Truth be told, depletion can even practically exist independent from anyone else with no hidden systemic issue. These may essentially show itself as the body's normal response to the accompanying unfortunate ways of life:

Inadequate eating routine

Bad sleeping paterns

Poor anxiety administration and work-life adjust

Mental despair

These are only the cases of option conclusions that have nothing to do with the endocrine framework. By then the examining doctor has effectively distinguished the wellspring of physical fatigue created by other irrelevant elements. Be that as it may, imagine a scenario where the underlying examinations (if done accurately) point the imperfection in the adrenaline glands showed by the lacking creation of cortisol.

25

Has the doctor officially found the tricky adrenal fatigue? One moment…

Ruling Out: Level Two

The past section clarified how the medical group is isolated in the adrenal fatigue debate. Contrasted with adrenal fatigue, Addison's Disease is a simpler issue to conclude in light of the fact that it is effectively unmistakable under solid medicinal examinations. Fundamentally, Addison's Disease is a harm in the adrenaline glands brought on by a fizzling safe framework. Inquisitively, this issue is regularly a result or a manifestation of other non-endocrine inadequacy. These are the accompanying genuine issue that outcome to Addison's Disease.

Cancer (e.g. lymphoma)

Advanced Immune Deficiency Syndrome (AIDS)

Tuberculosis

Observe: Addison's Disease is finished up by watching the harm in the adrenaline glands. Possibly either of the adrenaline glands swell, recoil, manage minor sores or secure other evident distortions. The primary contrast between this previously mentioned sickness and adrenal fatigue is that "the last's inadequate cortisol creation is not brought about by any natural harm". Curiously, Addison's Disease is not just constrained to the three common indications of physical mental and passionate weakness. Beside general exhaustion, these are the other after signs that hit the stamp for Addison's Disease:

Darkening pigment on the palm and joints

Dizziness after standing up

Lack of menstrual cycle for females

An ailment like adrenal fatigue is inclined to a false finding in view of the various components a doctor needs to preclude. It is regular for some specialists to just expect that identifying adrenal fatigue is only a "wild goose chase" not deserving of genuine consideration. In medieval circumstances, pharmacists would have made the same pretentious conclusion with respect to complex infections like tuberculosis because of the undeniable absence of information, innovation, and assets.

Top 10 Facts

Concerning test of recognizing adrenal fatigue, one ought to consider a comparable similarity as far as national security. Subsequently, in light of the fact that psychological militants are hard to find does not really mean they don't exist. In a simply logical universe of solution, wariness perseveres as a component in each possible strategy for examination until all conceivable disclosures are depleted.

Dr. Michael Lam is one of the main advocates of adrenal fatigue in the mid 90's.

While his contemporary, Dr. James Wilson, depicted the general way of this disputable infection, he has set down ten basic certainties that look to expose the common distrust managed against adrenal fatigue. Here are the accompanying "dynamic" clarifications defending the veracity of adrenal exhaustion:

1. Adrenal fatigue is real.

The principal adjust move in demonstrating a specific thought or idea is by guaranteeing it to be valid. One method for doing it is to give a strong definition. As indicated by Dr. Lam, adrenal fatigue is a problematic wellbeing connected to an accumulation of non-particular side effects.

2. Symptoms of adrenal fatigue are wide and varied.

Aside from the already said general weariness, there are other numerous particular manifestations to consider. These incorporate sleep deprivation, tension, low circulatory strain, muscle torment, et al. Basically, "distortion" is not generally precisely the most ideal approach to address a mind boggling issue.

3. Our understanding of adrenal fatigue is in its infancy.

In the same way as other clever researchers, Dr. Lam perceives the present restrictions of contemporary restorative innovation. By prudence of relationship, the absence of capacity to find a fear based oppressor doesn't mean he or she doesn't exist. It would be plain haughtiness to acknowledge that there is no more opportunity to get better in prescription.

4. Many of the symptoms of adrenal fatigue are hormone-related.

Since adrenal fatigue side effects are hormone-related, traditional types of treatment are intended to remedy the prompt inconvenience. In any case, straightforward concealment of the side effects regularly covers the basic condition that causes hormone unevenness. Consequently, customary types of treatment are a shallow technique that will undoubtedly bomb over the long haul.

5. Each person's biological constitution is unique.

Another sacred insight that Dr. Lam looks to grant is the intricacy of interesting individual physiology. In view of this, it is essentially indiscreet to finish up a specific issue in light of a wide range of responses from different patients. Some may show solid indications without adrenal exhaustion while others might experience the ill effects of adrenal fatigue without clear signs.

6. Adrenal fatigue crashes are real and unpleasant.

Adrenaline fatigue crashes happen toward the end of a quick reaction to upsetting conditions. This is brought about by the body's powerlessness to recoup rapidly from such responses. In extreme cases, a patient might be laid up after simply encountering a strained circumstance. The body returns to low vitality levels keeping in mind the end goal to "feel stable".

7. *Proper nutritional supplementation is necessary for recovery.*

By the descriptive word "legitimate", Dr. Lam recommends that utilization of wholesome supplements ought to be nearly observed as far as measurement and recurrence. The fundamental motivation behind why the endorsed medications blowback is basically on the grounds that patients are not subjected to long haul close supervision regarding controlling the treatment.

8. *Good exercise can help adrenal recovery, but it has to be accomplished correctly.*

Aside from nutritious supplements, another remedial measure that requires strict supervision is work out. As per Dr. Lam, a patient must not overexert or else it might trigger an adrenal fatigue crash. Fundamentally, a great practice must not instigate stress or weight. Above all, a great practice must be joined by a sound eating routine.

9. *The traditional blood test is not helpful.*

Not at all like other unending issue, a customary blood test is inapplicable in diagnosing adrenal fatigue. By goodness of similarity, one may contrast this strategy with stereotyping ethnic foundations so as to clarify an individual's identity. As Dr. Lam would put it, "a solitary depiction of one's hormonal capacity at one specific point in time from time to time recounts the entire story and, truth be told, might deceive.

10. The key to complete adrenal fatigue recovery lies in finding a highly experienced professional.

To the extent Dr. Lam is concerned, the most ideal approach to address adrenal fatigue (given the present phase of earliest stages as far as understanding this issue), is to grasp an all encompassing "personality body" approach. This involves a mix of eating routine, way of life modification and dietary supplements. Note: assist clarification about general treatment will be examined in Chapter 4 of this book.

Stages of Illness

It takes more than definition and straight actualities to set up the veracity of a specific disease. Advocates of the adrenal fatigue did not just infer that such issue is too genuine to reject, they have likewise soundly kept up that adrenal fatigue requests a lot of consideration.

Much the same as different genuine interminable ailments (e.g. Helps, tuberculosis, and disease), adrenal fatigue is a dynamic issue that is ordered under different stages. Here is the essential once-over of every stage, to a great extent in light of the shared research of the adrenal exhaustion examples:

Stage 1: Alarm Phase

This underlying phase of adrenal fatigue is frequently portrayed by gentle side effects of depletion. Given the trouble of setting up a reasonable examination in this stage, the caution stage now and again does not radiate clear indications specified in the previous two parts of this book. Fundamentally, the adrenaline organs work typically it could be said that it is still fit for creating a lot of hormones to adapt up to stressors.

Be that as it may, lab tests may uncover a relative increment in the levels of cortisol, epinephrine, androstenolone steroid (DHEA), and insulin. Generally, a man may encounter visit sharpness and energy. Thus, an individual is marginally more fomented than other ordinary individuals. As an immediate consequence of these sudden blasts of vitality, a man may experience the ill effects of unpredictable resting designs and exchanging tiredness.

Stage 2: Continuing Phase

Amid this stage, a more obvious hormonal awkwardness may occur. While the endocrine framework is still genuinely prepared to react to stressors, the ordinary level of sex hormones may start to disintegrate. Generally, the adrenaline glands are moderately unequipped for multitasking between empowering the body to adapt up to stretch and creating sex hormones. To the extent the body is concerned, the utility of self-protection outweighs everything else. These organs are creating more anxiety hormones and less sex hormones.

In light of the relative level of hormonal awkwardness, an individual experiencing stage 2 of adrenal fatigue may feel "wired but tired". For instance; in return for raised levels of mindfulness amid the daytime, he or she may encounter a drawn out depletion when the body's vitality level accidents during the evening. One particular sign is connected with overwhelming reliance on stimulants (e.g. espresso or chocolate bars) to support oneself all through whatever is left of the waking hours. Amid this stage, an individual may not really want to visit the specialist however certain examples may frequently stand out enough to be noticed.

Stage 3: Resistance Phase

At the point when the body achieves the Resistance Phase, the capacity of the adrenaline glands to deliver sex hormones is "completely" committed to the errand of creating stress hormones. Basically, the capacity to create testosterone and regular steroids (among others) is being delayed with a specific end goal to suit to the "chaotic" cortisol generation.

An individual may even now have the capacity to live regularly (e.g. clutch a vocation, keep up social connection with companions, or even perform fundamental routine errands). In any case, the personal satisfaction starts to weaken because of an absence of energy. It requires a noteworthy push to wind up distinctly sexually excited and, at more awful, sentimental connections may start to hint at limitation. Physically, the agony individual is routinely depleted and he or she may turn out to be more inclined to a few contaminations (e.g. regular influenza).

These arrangement of physical distresses might be a tad bit harder to address since they come to pass longer periods, some taking months while others anguishing them for a considerable length of time to come. Organize 3 is apparently the most conspicuous point of all periods of adrenal fatigue. It was frequently amid this phase individuals may start to look for legitimate counsel with specialists.

Stage 4: Burnout Phase

This phase of adrenal fatigue has as of now rendered the individual for all intents and purposes temperamental. Amid the Burnout Phase, the body's capacity to deliver both anxiety and sex hormones are achieving an unfaltering decay. Fundamentally, the body is gradually losing its ground as far as battling off anxiety.

An individual enduring experiencing stage 4 of adrenal fatigue is as of now overcome with extraordinary tiredness. Other physical inconveniences incorporate sudden weight reduction and more successive and delayed contaminations. Now and again, a man may likewise endure greatly poor memory. It requires a huge push to concentrate on one modest errand and it is much harder to get things finished. Thus, work execution turns out to be extremely poor and one might be at danger of losing business.

Getting sexually stimulated appeared like a far off adolescent memory. Mentally, a man experiencing this period of adrenal fatigue is likewise experiencing a much higher recurrence of hostile to social sessions. He or she will probably keep away from social collaboration and would frequently feel effortlessly fractious. A man achieving this stage is frequently discouraged, passionless and critical - overpowered by negative feelings. In most pessimistic scenarios, one may feel that life itself futile.

It is basic for people effectively enduring a phase 4 adrenal fatigue to look for quick assistance from experienced wellbeing experts. The degree of the treatment incorporates a total way of life change. Much the same as hypertension and other unending ailment, it is basically difficult to totally turn around the degree of harm done by the Burnout Phase in a given time allotment. It is conceivable to recuperate from such issue however it must be overseen even after the underlying manifestations are significantly lessened. Treatment involves a lifetime duty since serious manifestations may reemerge when the patient "takes his or her foot off the pedal"

Chapter 4: Treatment

As definitely clarified by the two past sections, adrenal fatigue is essentially a terrifying sickness. What makes it particularly guileful is that, as Dr. Lam would put it, our insight into this ailment is in its early stages. Medical science has scarcely touched the most superficial layer as far as thorough information concerning adrenal fatigue. The absence of data is certainly the most upsetting component in managing this issue. The way that there is no total accord among all individuals from the medical group concerning the veracity of adrenal fatigue as an illness basically outlines the desperate level of vulnerability.

However, an all-encompassing way to deal with a solid way of life has frequently withstood hundreds of years of examination as far as being a viable method for opposing infection – both genuine and envisioned. The agonizingly exhausted maxim "prevention is better than cure" couldn't be more sensible with regards to tending to a baffling issue like adrenal fatigue. By righteousness of relationship, ask yourself… Would you try knowing the identity of a potential assailant oblivious rear way rather than basically avoiding the territory?

Diet Restriction

Hippocrates, the Ancient Greek specialist, and Father of Western drug, cited an essential insight that is still broadly obeyed by present day social insurance guidelines today. He said, "Let your food be your medicine, and your medicine your food." Since the Classical Antiquities, the main line of mindful treatment involves picking a solid eating regimen. The infamous 21st Century push disorder called adrenal fatigue is no special case to this antiquated sacred run the show.

Expending the endorsed sustenances is similarly as similarly critical as maintaining a strategic distance from the taboo ones. The short way to picking your endorsed menu lies at the accompanying four hyphenated catchphrases: supplement rich, fiber-rich, low-sugar, and low-cholesterol.

With the end goal of highlighting a clearer abstain from food regimen, let us highlight the sorts of substances one must reject. These are the accompanying sustenance and drinks boycotted by adrenal weariness specialists:

Caffeine

Drinking espresso is not prudent to any individual who may have been experiencing adrenal fatigue. Stimulants disturb dozing designs and initiate pressure, hence upsetting the capacity of the adrenaline glands to recuperate from inordinate discharge of cortisol. On the off chance that juiced refreshments are unavoidable, it ought to be overwhelmed by strict control amid daytime.

Sugar and Artificial Sweeteners

Devouring an excess of sugar has been a guilty party to a wide assortment of wellbeing intricacies, especially diabetes and hypertension. A similar standard applies to adrenal fatigue administration since hyperglycemia tends to annoy the characteristic adjust of cortisol and different anxiety hormones. Raw nectar and stevia are more prudent other option to adding sweet flavor to one's sustenance.

Processed & Microwaved Foods

The primary motivation behind why prepared and microwaved sustenance are prohibited for individuals suspected or determined to have adrenal fatigue has a great deal to do with assimilation. Nourishments with fillers and additives take a more huge volume of vitality to separate. To the extent managing adrenal fatigue is concerned, a man must have the capacity to advance his or her vitality levels, not bargain it. It is more desirable over eat entire meat sources like chicken, turkey and greasy fish for a considerable wellspring of protein and minerals. Nuts, seeds, and vegetables are likewise essential.

Hydrogenated Oils

Individuals who may have adrenal fatigue should likewise stay away from vegetable oils. An exceptionally ignitable substance like hydrogenated oils may prompt to adrenal irritation. A more appropriate option for greasy eating regimen incorporate olive oil, coconut oil, and natural margarine.

Supplements

Ordinarily, eating the correct nourishment is sufficient to maintain a more strong and versatile body. Lamentably, eras of poor cultivating hones have encouraged a biological system that bargained the nature of products and domesticated animals. Vegetables are developed in engineered medium, if not tainted soil. Cultivate creatures subsist on substandard scavenge. Consequently, the great wellsprings of supplements may not stack up to the ideal needs of a body tormented by adrenal exhaustion.

Thus, nutritious supplements were produced to address a wide assortment of dietary inadequacies. Taking the accompanying supplements can oversee adrenal fatigue:

- Vitamin C
- Vitamin B5
- Vitamin B12
- Vitamin D3
- Magnesium
- Zinc
- DHA (Fish oils)

- ☐ Holy basil
- ☐ Indian ginseng

Lifestyle Adjustments

There's a whole other world to wellbeing than the stuff individuals put in their bodies. Truth be told, standards, individual propensities, and environment assume a critical part in maintaining wellbeing. On the off chance that normal individuals are required to carry on with a solid way of life, a more noteworthy arrangement of consideration is involved in upgrading the general state of individuals who may have adrenal fatigue. It makes sense that anxiety is an indistinguishable component in life. All the better you can do is to minimize your general introduction to upsetting conditions.

Rest when you feel tired as much as possible.

Listen to your body. Tiredness is a characteristic reaction of the body to recharge its vitality. One needs to recognize that fighting the temptation to rest in times of depletion is basically an oblivious type of causing self-hurt. Sadly, individuals abstain from inexhaustible lay on records of ordinarily misjudged hard working attitudes (e.g. "a gainful individual is an exhausted machine").

Maintain 8 to 10 hours of daily sleep.

The body requires a normal of 8 to 10 hours of rest for every day. In any case, knowing the correct time to resign during the evening is considerably more vital than basically snoozing all through the recommended length. Abstain from remaining up late on a general rest cycle so as not to strain your ordinary vitality levels.

Eat at the right time, frequency and volume.

Aside from the prior counsel to share a sound supper, it is much more essential to observe the time one chooses to eat. For example, a 12-hour hole amongst breakfast and the following supper is an unfortunate eating routine practice that tend to bring about gorging – vanquishing the whole motivation behind the solid eating routine program. Eating at the correct time creates a positive domino impact. Consequently, there is little need to expand the substance allow as an aftereffect of taking suppers too soon or past the point of no return than the planned timetable.

Exercise according to your own pace.

Despite the fact that overexertion can jeopardize a man suspected with adrenal fatigue, latency will leave his or her insufficient anxiety hormone generation stagnant. Unfaltering activity will permit for all intents and purposes every crucial organ to step by step enhance (considering that there is no hidden uncertain damage). Observe: Listen to your brain and body. On the off chance that a specific physical action (paying little

41

heed to the level of effort) no more drawn out "triggers a solid reward framework", the time has come to stop. There is nothing more hindering than working out and feeling horrible in view of driving oneself to a limit. There's a tremendous contrast between doing work out and getting worked up.

Always seek the positive side of life.

In the specific instance of adrenal weariness, the normal proverb "chuckling is the best medication" is basically too great to be an adage. At the point when an individual is suffused with positive vibes, he or she has a superior possibility of saving and streamlining vitality. Generally, lesser uneasiness implies a lesser requirement for the adrenaline glands to create stretch hormones. Positive vibes adequately evacuate the possibility to open oneself to nervousness.

Seek counseling or support if it's hard.

Given that countless in the lay and restorative group have acknowledged adrenal fatigue as a genuine disease, it makes sense that no one ought to need to manage this issue alone. A man can just do as such much with his or her own particular exertion, assurance and activity. Be that as it may, the odds of prevailing in this attempt will duplicate with an exceptionally powerful emotionally supportive network. Being encompassed by individuals who will support your advance gives you the one thing anyone could seldom obtain all alone - motivation to keep living

Conclusion

Another day has touched base as you briskly inspired yourself up from the bed. You strolled energetically to the lavatory to exhaust your bladders. In the wake of soothing yourself, you took a gander at the clock that showed 6:00 AM. You didn't require a wake up timer since you've as of now hit the sack at 9:30 PM.

It is an excellent Saturday morning, and the whole seven occupied weekdays didn't somewhat abandon you worn out. You gave and wiped yourself dry. At that point you put on your adaptable track pants, hoody coat, and running shoes. After quickly extending your appendages, you hit the street in long walks for a 3-mile run. The charming odor of the morning dew lingered palpably, and you are filling your lungs with each floating breeze of it.

You arrived home almost an hour after your workout, sweat-doused and somewhat sore everywhere on your legs. After your second shower, you set up your breakfast: two bits of crisp veggie sandwich, five cuts of oranges, and some sweet-noticing ginseng tea. A sound without caffeine breakfast is a decent approach to renew your vitality after a charming outside work out.

In the wake of completing four sections of the dream book you obtained from the general

43

population library the previous evening, you concluded that it's a great opportunity to accomplish something gainful following a couple of hours of insightful stimulation. So you spruced up, took off of the house and strolled the distance to the recreation center to take photos of the forcing scene. You have likewise chosen to walk the distance to the wharf and take a preview of the beautiful red blasting nightfall in the sea-going skyline. Today is a lovely day, and you plan to end it with a sentimental date at a road side bistro by sunset. Force, uplifting viewpoint and the unquenchable energy forever were the astonishing highlights of your day.

The past story appeared like a long ways from the presentation, would it say it isn't? Sounds like a story-book meaning of a solid and cheerful way of life. In any case, it becomes anybody with a firm handle of reality that not all days could be as wired and as impeccable as the hypothetical storyline in the past indisputable passages. There is no mischief in perceiving the substances of stress, weariness, and strain in life. Awful days are will undoubtedly happen, even in your treasured ends of the week.

Be that as it may, there is a complete line between constant unfortunate despondency and incidental snapshots of wretchedness. By acclimatizing yourself to a solid way of life, your body is adapted for a more positive demeanor. In the event that you are enthusiastic, you will feel more slanted to play out any movement with a solid drive for perfection. You are more avid to gain from hands-on involvement, paying little mind to regardless of whether it would deliver the coveted result. It will even take somewhat more than a disagreeable incitement (e.g. being pestered by a more bizarre driving by) to destroy half of your day. On the off chance that you are steadily wellbeing cognizant, the general nature of your life will be a ton better.

As a mainstream (antique) saying may put it, "wellbeing is riches". Subsequent to finding out about the potential threats of adrenal fatigue, you may be more disposed to concur that "health is the only wealth". Your physical condition influences every single other part of your life. It is just fitting to protect it with a lot of enthusiasm, criticalness, and carefulness.

References:

Wilson, James L., MD. "Frequently Asked Questions on Adrenal Fatigue." Adrenal Fatigue. Future Formulations, LLC, n.d. Web. 16 Sept. 2016.

"What Is the Adrenal Gland?" Organs of the Body. N.p., n.d. Web. 16 Sept. 2016.

Wilson, James L., MD. "Dr. Wilson's Burnout Questionnaire." Adrenal Fatigue. Future Formulations, LLC, n.d. Web. 16 Sept. 2016.

Metcalf, Eric, MPH, and Brunilda Nazario, MD. "Adrenal Fatigue: Symptoms, Causes, Treatment." WebMD. WebMD, n.d. Web. 16 Sept. 2016.

Axe, Josh, DC. "3 Steps to Heal Adrenal Fatigue Naturally - Dr. Axe." Dr Axe. Kymera, 29 June 2016. Web. 16 Sept. 2016.

"Myth vs. Fact." Adrenal Fatigue Myth vs Fact. Endocrine Society, n.d. Web. 16 Sept. 2016.

"Adrenal Insufficiency and Addison's Disease." U.S National Library of Medicine. National Institute of Diabetes and Digestive and Kidney Diseases, n.d. Web. 16 Sept. 2016.

Gavura, Scott. "Fatigued by a Fake Disease." Science-Based Medicine, 28 Oct. 2010. Web. 16 Sept. 2016.

Hansen, Fawne. "Adrenal Fatigue: A Controversial Diagnosis?" Adrenal Fatigue Solution. Perfect Health, n.d. Web. 16 Sept. 2016.

Hansen, Fawne. "The Four Stages of Adrenal Fatigue." Adrenal Fatigue Solution. Perfect Health, n.d. Web. 16 Sept. 2016.

Hansen, Fawne. "The History of Adrenal Fatigue." Adrenal Fatigue Solution. Perfect Health, n.d. Web. 16 Sept. 2016.

Garrett, Cindy Lynn. "Top 10 Adrenal Fatigue Facts Made Easy." Dr. Lam Body Mind Nutrition. N.p., n.d. Web. 16 Sept. 2016.